Diabetic
Air Fryer Recipes

Prepare Delicious Easy-to-Make Recipes to Boost Your Energy and Health

Lilith Ballard

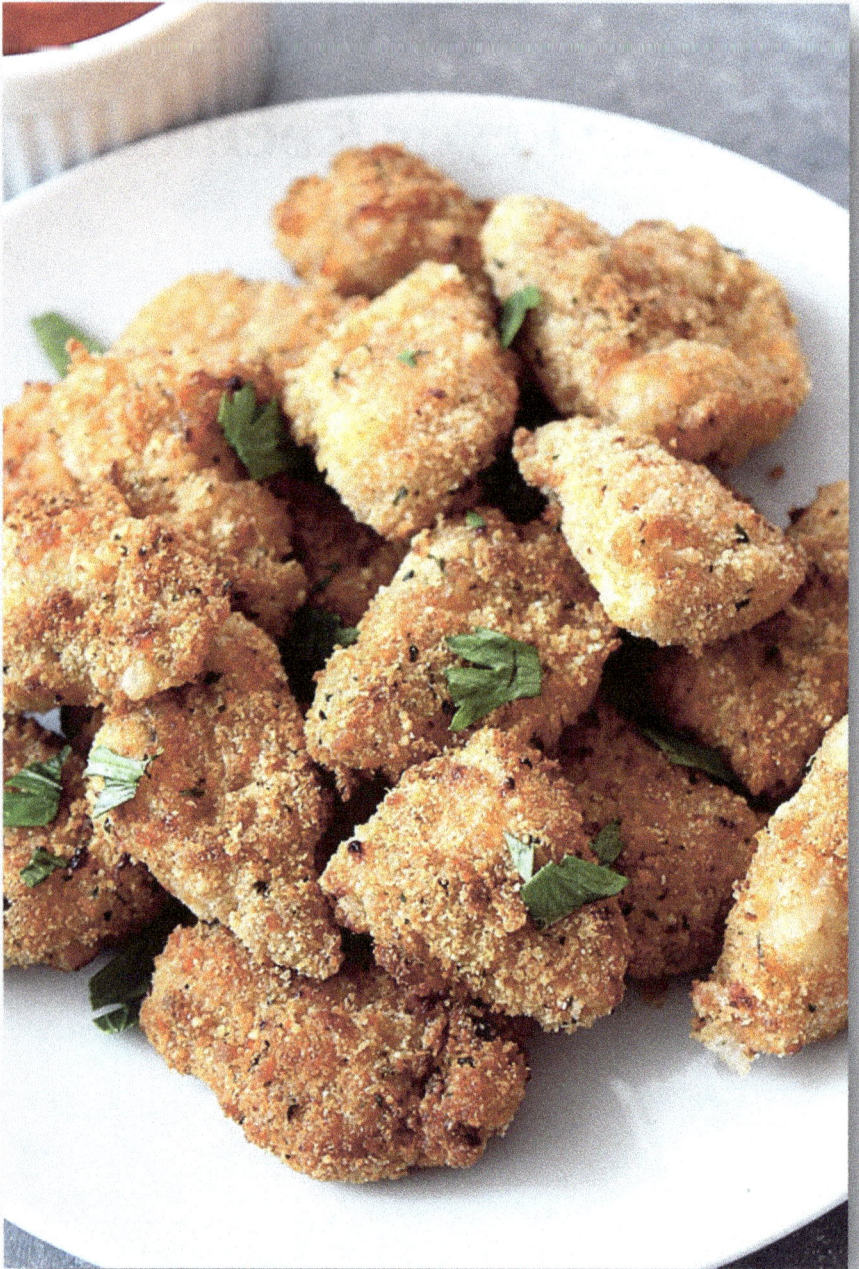

professional before attempting any techniques outlined in this book.

by reading this document, the reader agrees that under no circumstances is the author responsible for any losses, direct or indirect, which are incurred as a result of the use of information contained within this document, including, but not limited to, — errors, omissions, or inaccuracies.

Table of Contents

AIR FRYER TOFU

Preparation Time: 45 minutes

Cooking Time: 10 minutes

Servings: 1

Nutritional values:

- Calories: 115 kcal
- Fat: 4 g
- Carbohydrates: 2 g
- Proteins: 7 g

Ingredients:

- 16 oz. block added company tofu.
- 2 tbsp. Low salt soy sauce.
- 1 tbsp. additional virgin olive oil.
- 1 tsp. diced garlic.
- ½ tsp. sriracha.
-

Directions:

1. Press Tofu-Use a tofu press, or line a plate with paper towels. Place a block of tofu ahead as well as place more

paper towels on the top of the tofu so that the tofu is sandwiched between paper towels. Place a heavy pan on top of the tofu with 4 hefty containers in addition to the pan. Enable to sit for thirty minutes.

2. When tofu is pushed cut into 1-inch dices.

3. Mix soy sauce, olive oil, garlic, as well as sriracha in a small bowl. Turn tofu halfway with marinating time to make sure all sides saturate up the sauce.

4. Set tofu in the air fryer basket in a single layer. Don't jam-pack. Cook for 10 minutes at 375°F. Toss at the 5-minute mark.

AIR FRYER ASPARAGUS

Preparation Time: 3 minutes

Cooking Time: 10 minutes

Servings: 1

Nutritional values:

- Calories: 31 kcal
- Fat: 3 g
- Carbohydrates: 0 g
- Proteins: 0.2 g

Ingredients:

- 1 tbsp. olive oil.
- 1 package of asparagus spears.
- Seasoning your choice.

Directions:

1.   Tidy your asparagus spears by running them under cool water in your kitchen sink, taking off any particles from your spears. You can utilize a vegetable clean here if you have that accessible.

2.   Cut the white thick stalky ends off of your asparagus spears with a sharp blade, leaving only the environment-friendly spears, heads still connected.

3.   Set the cleansed and reduced spears in the bottom of your air fryer and drizzle with 1 tbsp. of olive oil. Using a basting brush, spread out the olive oil evenly over the asparagus.

4.   Sprinkle with your preferred seasonings, and after that, air fry for 10 minutes at 380°F. Remove from heat and serve.

AIR FRYER BRUSSELS SPROUTS

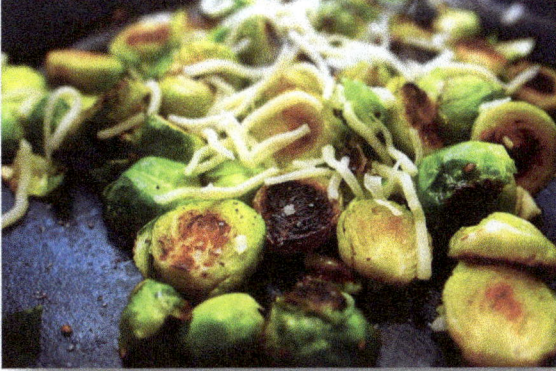

Preparation Time: 15 minutes

Cooking Time: 18 minutes

Servings: 1

Nutritional values:

- Calories: 50 kcal
- Fat: 4 g
- Carbohydrates: 4 g
- Proteins: 1 g

Ingredients:

- 2 cups halved brussels sprouts
- 1 tbsp. olive oil.
- ¼ tsp. sea salt.

Directions:

1. Preheat the air fryer to 375°F for 5 minutes.
2. Toss the sprouts in a bowl with olive oil as well as add to the air fryer.
3. Gently spray the basket with olive oil cooking spray. Add the sprouts and also cook for 9 minutes or to your desired level of crunchy.
4. Salt finished sprouts to taste.

AIR FRYER ROASTED GARLIC

Preparation Time: 5 minutes

Cooking Time: 31 minutes

Servings: 1

Nutritional values:

- Calories: 31 kcal
- Fat: 1 g
- Carbohydrates: 5 g
- Proteins: 1 g

Ingredients:

- 2 heads garlic.
- 1 tsp. olive oil.

Directions:

1. Cut the tops off of the garlic heads, exposing the specific cloves.

2. Arrange the bulbs in the middle of an item of foil and drizzle olive oil over the garlic bulbs' tops. Pro pointer: the amount of olive oil required will depend on the dimension of garlic heads you are making use of.

3. Tightly finish up the garlic in the aluminum foil and location in the basket of your air fryer.

4. Cook for 27 minutes at 400°F.

5. The delicately browns the top of the light bulbs.

BLISTERED SHISHITO PEPPERS

Preparation Time: 5 minutes

Cooking Time: 11 minutes

Servings: 2

Nutritional values:

- Calories: 32 kcal
- Fat: 1 g
- Carbohydrates: 5 g
- Proteins: 0.1 g

Ingredients:

- 1 lb. Shishito peppers washed as well as pat dry.
- 1 tsp. sesame oil.
- ¼ tsp. coconut amino.
- Kosher salt.
- Sesame seeds

Directions:

1. Put the peppers in the basket of your air fryer and spray with olive oil food preparation.

2. Prepare at 350°F for 10 minutes, trembling the basket midway. Food preparation time will depend on your peppers' size and how "done" you desire them.

3. Add the peppers to a bowl with the sesame oil and coconut amino.

WHOLE WHEAT PIZZAS IN AN AIR FRYER

Preparation Time: 10 minutes

Cooking Time: 8 minutes

Servings: 4

Nutritional values:

- Calories: 229 kcal
- Fat: 5 g
- Carbohydrates: 2 g
- Proteins: 11 g

Ingredients:

- 2 whole-wheat pita rounds
- ¼ ounce shaved Parmigiano-Reggiano cheese (about 1 tbsp.)
- ¼ cup lower-sodium marinara sauce
- 1 small plum tomato
- 1 small garlic clove, thinly sliced

- 1 ounce pre-shredded part-skim mozzarella cheese (about ¼ cup)
- 1 cup baby spinach leaves (1 oz.)

Directions:

1. Cut the tomato into 8 slices.
2. Spread the marinara sauce on 1 side of each of the pita bread. Ensure you spread the sauce evenly.
3. Top the bread with cheese, garlic, tomato slices, and spinach leaves.
4. Place the pita bread in your air fryer. Set the temperature to 350°F and heat the bread for about 5 minutes. This will melt the cheese completely. Do this to every piece of pita bread.
5. You can then serve them.

QUICK FRY CHICKEN WITH CAULIFLOWER

Preparation Time: 5 minutes

Cooking Time: 18 minutes

Servings: 4

Nutritional values:

- Calories: 220 kcal
- Fat: 9 g
- Carbohydrates: 13.6 g
- Proteins: 30.5 g

Ingredients:

For the quick fry:

- 1½ pounds chicken thigh fillets, diced
- 1 piece, small red bell pepper, julienned
- 1 piece, thumb-sized ginger, grated

- 2 tbsp. olive oil
- 1 clove, large garlic, minced
- 2 stalks, large leeks, minced
- 1 can, 5 oz. water chestnuts, quartered
- 1 head, small cauliflower, cut into bite-sized florets
- ¾ cups chicken stock, low sodium

Seasonings:

- 1 tsp. stevia
- 1 tbsp. fish sauce
- ½ tbsp. cornstarch, dissolved in
- 4 tbsp. water
- Pinch salt
- Pinch black pepper, to taste

Garnish:

- Leeks, minced
- 1 large lime, cut into 6 wedges

Directions:

1. Preheat Air Fryer to 330°F.
2. Pour olive oil in a pan. Swirl pan to coat. Sauté garlic, ginger, and leeks for 2 minutes. Set aside. Add in water chestnuts, cauliflower, red bell pepper, and chicken broth. Stir well. Cook for 15 minutes.

3. Meanwhile, put the chicken in the air fryer basket. Fry until seared and golden brown.

4. Add seasoning into the pan. Stir and cook until the juice thickens.

5. Ladle 1 portion of quick fry veggies and chicken, Garnish with leeks and lemon wedges on the side. Serve.

ARTICHOKE HEARTS

Preparation Time: 5 minutes

Cooking Time: 8 minutes

Servings: 3

Nutritional values:

- Calories: 67 kcal
- Fat: 3 g
- Carbohydrates: 7 g
- Proteins: 2 g

Ingredients:

- 1 pound frozen artichoke hearts, thawed, quartered
- 1 cup plain yogurt, low fat
- 2 eggs, whisked
- 1 cup almond flour, finely milled
- 1 cup almond flour, coarsely milled
- 1 small lime, sliced into wedges, pips removed
- ½ cup sour cream, reduced-fat
- Pinch sea salt

Directions:

1. Preheat Air Fryer to 330°F.

2. In a bowl, combine yogurt and salt. Soak artichoke hearts for 15 minutes. Drain. Discard yogurt.

3. Dredge artichokes in almond flour first, then into eggs, and into coarse-milled almond flour.

4. Layer artichoke hearts into the Air Fryer basket. Fry for 5 minutes or until golden brown on all sides. Drain on paper towels. Squeeze lime juice. Serve with lime wedges and sour cream on the side.

AIR-FRYER ONION STRINGS

Preparation Time: 15 minutes

Cooking Time: 8 minutes

Servings: 4

Nutritional values:

- Calories: 150 kcal
- Fat: 17 g
- Carbohydrates: 13 g
- Proteins: 2 g

Ingredients:

- 2 cups buttermilk
- 1 piece, whole white onion, halved, julienned
- 2 cups almond flour, finely milled
- ½ tsp. cayenne pepper
- Pinch sea salt
- Pinch black pepper to taste

Directions:

1. Preheat Air Fryer to 330°F.

2. Soak onion strings in buttermilk for 1 hour before frying. Drain.

3. Meanwhile, mix almond flour, cayenne pepper, salt, and pepper in a bowl. Coat onion strings with flour mixture.

4. Layer onions in the air fryer basket. Fry until golden brown and crisp. Drain on paper towels. Season with salt. Serve.

FRIED SPINACH

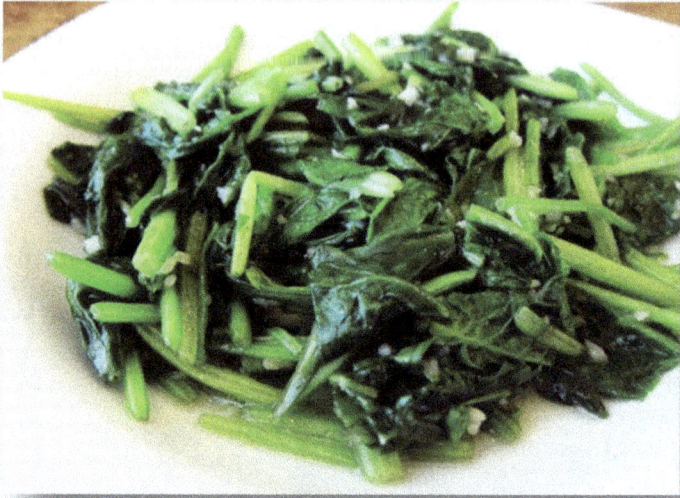

Preparation Time: 14 minutes

Cooking Time: 5 minutes

Servings: 3

Nutritional values:

- Calories: 81.6
- Fat: 6.9 g
- Carbohydrates: 4.5 g
- Proteins: 1.3 g

Ingredients:

- 2½ pounds fresh spinach leaves and tender stems only
- Pinch sea salt, to taste

Directions:

1. Preheat Air Fryer to 330°F.
2. Put spinach in the Air fryer basket. Fry for 20 seconds. Drain on paper towels. Repeat the step with the rest of the spinach. Season with salt. Serve.

ZUCCHINI FLOWERS

Preparation Time: 14 minutes

Cooking Time: 10 minutes

Servings: 3

Nutritional values:

- Calories: 117 kcal
- Fat: 8 g
- Carbohydrates: 8 g
- Proteins: 1 g

Ingredients:

- 2½ pounds zucchini flowers, rinsed
- 1 cup almond flour, finely milled
- Pinch sea salt, to taste
- Balsamic vinegar, for garnish

Directions:

1. Preheat Air Fryer to 330°F.

2.   Half-fill deep fryer with oil. Set this at medium heat. Lightly season zucchini flowers with salt, and then dredge in almond flour.

3.   Layer breaded flowers into the Air Fryer basket. Fry until golden brown. Drain on paper towels. Transfer to a plate. Pour balsamic vinegar if using. Serve.

GARLIC BREAD WITH CHEESE DIP

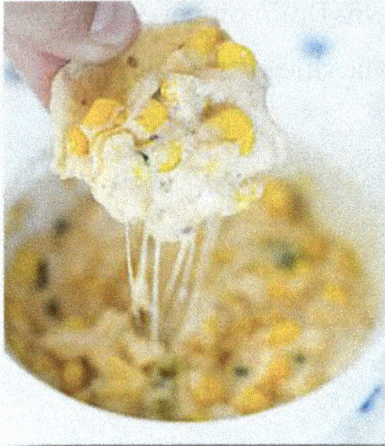

Preparation Time: 8 minutes

Cooking Time: 16 minutes

Servings: 8

Nutritional values:

- Calories: 209
- Fat: 8 g
- Carbohydrates: 29 g
- Proteins: 2.9 g

Ingredients:

Fried garlic bread:

- 1 medium baguette, halved lengthwise, cut sides toasted
- 2 garlic cloves, whole
- 4 tbsp. extra virgin olive oil
- 2 tbsp. fresh parsley, minced

Blue cheese dip:

- 1 Tbsp. fresh parsley, minced
- ¼ cup fresh chives, minced
- ¼ tsp. Tabasco sauce
- 1 tbsp. lemon juice, freshly squeezed
- ½ cup Greek yogurt, low fat
- ¼ cup blue cheese, reduced fat
- 1/16 tsp. salt
- 1/16 tsp. white pepper

Directions:

1. Preheat machine to 400°F.
2. Combine oil and parsley in a small bowl.
3. Vigorously rub garlic cloves on cut/toasted sides of the baguette. Dispose of garlic nubs.
4. Using a pastry brush, spread parsley-infused oil on the cut side of the bread.

5. Place bread cut-side down on a chopping board. Slice into inch-thick half-moons.
6. Place bread slices in the air Fryer basket. Fry for 3 to 5 minutes or until bread browns a little. Shake contents of basket once midway through. Place cooked pieces on a serving platter. Repeat the step for the remaining bread.
7. To prepare blue cheese dip: mix ingredients in a bowl.
8. Place equal portions of fried bread on plates. Serve with blue cheese dip on the side.

FRIED MIXED VEGGIES WITH AVOCADO DIP

Preparation Time: 9 minutes

Cooking Time: 11 minutes

Servings: 4

Nutritional values:

- Calories: 109
- Fat: 2.6 g
- Carbohydrates: 4.0 g
- Proteins: 2.9 g

Ingredients:

- Oil for spraying

Avocado-feta dip:

- 1 avocado, pitted, peeled, flesh scooped out
- 4 oz. feta cheese, reduced fat
- 2 leeks, minced

- 1 lime, freshly squeezed
- ¼ cup fresh parsley, chopped roughly
- 1/16 tsp. black pepper
- 1/16 tsp. salt

Vegetables:

- 1 zucchini, sliced into matchsticks
- 1 carrot, sliced into matchsticks
- 1 cup panko breadcrumbs, add more if needed
- 1 parsnip, sliced into matchsticks
- 1 large egg, whisked, add more if needed
- 1 cup all-purpose flour, add more if needed
- 1/8 tsp. flaky sea salt

Directions:

1. Preheat the Air Fryer to 400°F.
2. Season carrots, parsnips, and zucchini with salt.
3. Dredge carrots into flour first, then egg, and finally into breadcrumbs. Place breaded pieces on a baking sheet lined with parchment paper. Repeat the step for all the carrots. Then do the same for parsnips and zucchini.
4. Lightly spray vegetables with oil. Place a generous handful of carrots in the Air Fryer basket. Fry for 10 minutes or until breading turns golden brown, shaking contents of the

basket once midway. Place cooked pieces on a plate. Repeat the step for the remaining carrots.

5. Do the earlier step for parsnips, and then zucchini.

6. For the dip, except for salt, place the remaining ingredients in a food processor. Pulse a couple of times, and then process to desired consistency scraping down sides of the machine often. Taste. Add salt only if needed. Place in an airtight container. Chill until needed.

7. Place equal portions of cooked vegetables on plates. Serve with a small amount of avocado-feta dip on the side.

PHYLLO VEGETABLE TRIANGLES

Preparation Time: 15 minutes

Cooking Time: 6 to 11 minutes

Servings: 6

Nutritional values:

- Calories: 67
- Fat: 2 g
- Carbohydrates: 11 g
- Proteins: 2 g

Ingredients:

- 3 tbsp. minced onion
- 2 garlic cloves, minced
- 2 tbsp. grated carrot
- 1 tsp. olive oil
- 3 tbsp. frozen baby peas, thawed

- 2 tbsp. nonfat cream cheese, at room temperature
- 6 sheets frozen Phyllo dough, thawed
- Olive oil spray for coating the dough

Directions:

1. In a baking pan, combine the onion, garlic, carrot, and olive oil. Air fry at 390°F (199°C) for 2 to 4 minutes, or until the vegetables are crisp-tender. Transfer to a bowl.

2. Stir in the peas and cream cheese to the vegetable mixture. Let it cool while you prepare the dough.

3. Lay one sheet of phyllo on a work surface and lightly spray with olive oil spray. Top with another sheet of phyllo. Repeat with the remaining 4 phyllo sheets; you'll have 3 stacks with 2 layers each. Cut each stack lengthwise into 4 strips (12 strips total).

4. Place a scant 2 tsp. of the filling near the bottom of each strip. Bring one corner up over the filling to make a triangle; continue folding the triangles over, as you would fold a flag. Seal the edge with a bit of water. Repeat with the remaining strips and filling.

5. Air fry the triangles, in 2 batches, for 4 to 7 minutes or until golden brown. Serve.

RED CABBAGE AND MUSHROOM POT STICKERS

Preparation Time: 12 minutes

Cooking Time: 11–18 minutes

Servings: 12

Nutritional values:

- Calories: 88 kcal
- Fat: 3 g
- Carbohydrates: 14 g
- Proteins: 2 g

Ingredients:

- 1 cup shredded red cabbage
- ¼ cup chopped button mushrooms
- ¼ cup grated carrot
- 2 tbsp. minced onion
- 2 garlic cloves, minced
- 2 tsp. grated fresh ginger

- 12 gyoza/pot sticker wrappers
- 2½ tsp. olive oil, divided

Directions:

1. In a baking pan, combine the red cabbage, mushrooms, carrot, onion, garlic, and ginger. Add 1 tbsp. of water. Place in the Air Fryer and bake at 370°F (188°C) for 3 to 6 minutes, until the vegetables are crisp-tender. Drain and set aside.

2. Working one at a time, place the potsticker wrappers on a work surface. Top each wrapper with a scant 1 tbsp. of the filling. Fold half of the wrapper over the other half to form a half-circle. Dab one edge with water and press both edges together.

3. To the baking pan, add 1¼ tsp. of olive oil. Put half of the potstickers, seam-side up, in the pan. Air fry for 5 minutes, or until the bottoms are light golden brown. Add 1 tbsp. of water and return the pan to the Air Fryer.

4. Air fry for 4 to 6 minutes more, or until hot. Repeat with the remaining potstickers, remaining 1¼ tsp. of oil, and another tbsp. of water. Serve immediately.

GARLIC ROASTED MUSHROOMS

Preparation Time: 3 minutes

Cooking Time: 22–27 minutes

Servings: 4

Nutritional values:

- Calories: 128 kcal
- Fat: 4 g
- Carbohydrates: 17 g
- Proteins: 13 g

Ingredients:

- 16 garlic cloves, peeled
- 2 tsp. olive oil, divided
- 16 button mushrooms
- ½ tsp. dried marjoram
- 1/8 tsp. freshly ground black pepper
- 1 tbsp. white wine or low-sodium vegetable broth

Directions:

1. In a baking pan, mix the garlic with 1 tsp. of olive oil. Roast in the Air Fryer at 350°F (177°C) for 12 minutes.

2. Add the mushrooms, marjoram, and pepper. Stir to coat. Drizzle with the remaining 1 tsp. of olive oil and the white wine.

3. Return to the Air Fryer and roast for 10 to 15 minutes more, or until the mushrooms and garlic cloves are tender. Serve.

BAKED SPICY CHICKEN MEATBALLS

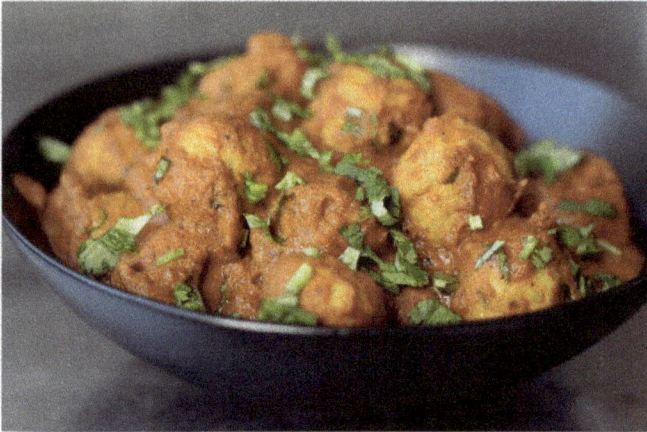

Preparation Time: 10 minutes

Cooking Time: 11–14 minutes

Servings: 24

Nutritional values:

- Calories: 186
- Fat: 7 g
- Carbohydrates: 5 g
- Proteins: 29 g

Ingredients:

- 1 medium red onion, minced
- 2 garlic cloves, minced
- 1 jalapeño pepper, minced
- 2 tsp. olive oil
- 3 tbsp. ground almonds
- 1 egg
- 1 tsp. dried thyme
- 1 pound (454 g) of ground chicken breast

Directions:

1. In a baking pan, combine the red onion, garlic, jalapeño, and olive oil. Bake at 400°F (204°C) for 3 to 4 minutes, or until the vegetables are crisp-tender. Transfer to a medium bowl.

2. Mix in the almonds, egg, and thyme to the vegetable mixture. Add the chicken and mix until just combined.

3. Form the chicken mixture into about 24 (1-inch) balls. Bake the meatballs, in batches, for 8 to 10 minutes until the chicken reaches an internal temperature of 165°F (74°C) on a meat thermometer.

MINI ONION BITES

Preparation Time: 10 minutes

Cooking Time: 16–20 minutes

Servings: 20

Nutritional values:

- Calories: 166 kcal
- Fat: 2 g
- Carbohydrates: 31 g
- Proteins: 6 g

Ingredients:

- 20 white boiler onions
- 1 cup buttermilk
- 2 eggs
- 1 cup flour
- 1 cup whole-wheat bread crumbs
- 1 tbsp. smoked paprika
- 1 tsp. salt
- 1 tsp. ground black pepper

- 1 tsp. granulated garlic
- ¾ tsp. chili powder
- Olive oil spray

Directions:

1. Place a parchment liner in the Air Fryer basket.
2. Slice off the root end of the onions, taking off as little as possible.
3. Peel off the papery skin and make cuts halfway through the tops of the onions. Don't cut too far down; you want the onion to hold together still.
4. In a large bowl, beat the buttermilk and eggs together.
5. In a medium bowl, mix the flour, bread crumbs, paprika, salt, pepper, garlic, and chili powder.
6. Add the prepared onions to the buttermilk mixture and allow to soak for at least 10 minutes.
7. Working in batches, remove the onions from the batter and dredge them with the bread crumb mixture.
8. Place the prepared onions in the Air Fryer basket in a single layer.
9. Spray lightly with the olive oil and air fry at 360°F (182°C) for 8 to 10 minutes, until golden and crispy. Repeat with any remaining onions and serve.

CRISPY PARMESAN CAULIFLOWER

Preparation Time: 12 minutes

Cooking Time: 14 to 17 minutes

Servings: 20

Nutritional values:

- Calories: 106 kcal
- Fat: 6 g
- Carbohydrates: 10 g
- Proteins: 3 g

Ingredients:

- 4 cups cauliflower florets
- 1 cup whole-wheat bread crumbs
- 1 tsp. coarse sea salt or kosher salt
- ¼ cup grated Parmesan cheese
- ¼ cup butter

- ¼ cup mild hot sauce
- Olive oil spray

Directions:

1. Place a parchment liner in the Air Fryer basket.

2. Cut the cauliflower florets in half and set them aside.

3. In a small bowl, mix the bread crumbs, salt, and Parmesan; set aside.

4. In a small microwave-safe bowl, combine the butter and hot sauce. Heat in the microwave until the butter is melted, about 15 seconds. Whisk.

5. Holding the stems of the cauliflower florets, dip them in the butter mixture to coat. Shake off any excess mixture.

6. Dredge the dipped florets with the bread crumb mixture, then put them in the Air Fryer basket. There's no need for a single layer; just toss them all in there.

7. Spray the cauliflower lightly with olive oil and air fry at 350°F (177°C) for 14 to 17 minutes, shaking the basket a few times throughout the cooking process. The florets are done when they are lightly browned and crispy. Serve warm.

GARLIC PARMESAN AIR FRYER ASPARAGUS

Preparation Time: 11 minutes

Cooking Time: 10-15 minutes

Servings: 4

Nutritional values:

- Calories: 56
- Fat: 3.7 g
- Carbohydrates: 4.9 g
- Proteins: 2.7 g

Ingredients:

- 1 pound asparagus
- 1 tsp. garlic powder
- 1 tbsp. olive oil
- 1 tbsp. grated parmesan
- Pinch kosher salt
- Dash pepper

Directions:

1.	Prepare the asparagus by cutting the bottom at least one or two inches.

2.	Transfer the asparagus slices on a tray or plate and then drizzle all over with olive oil.

3.	Sprinkle all over with garlic powder, grated cheese, and season with pepper and salt.

4.	Using your clean hands, toss the asparagus to coat thoroughly.

5.	Transfer the asparagus to the air fryer basket and cook for ten minutes at 400°F. Serve hot!

BEEF PATTY

Preparation Time: 9 minutes

Cooking Time: 33 minutes

Servings: 4

Nutritional values:

- Calories: 269 kcal
- Fat: 3.41 g
- Carbohydrates: 0 g
- Proteins: 20.9 g

Ingredients:

- Prepared dough
- 300g beef
- 1 large onion
- 1 red pepper
- 2 hard-boiled eggs
- Salt

- Pepper to taste.
- 1 tsp. oil

Directions:

1. Remove the dough from the refrigerator 10 minutes before.
2. In a pan, place oil, 1 onion, 1 pepper, garlic, seasoning. Add ground beef until cooked well. Season with salt and pepper to taste.
3. Let the filling cool
4. Place the filling in each circle of the dough and seal with egg white at the edges.
5. Butter a refractory mold and accommodate the patty.
6. Preheat the oven to 190°C for 10 minutes by pressing the Convection button
7. Place the refractory on the metal rack and bring it to the preheated oven for 30 minutes at 190°C.

AIR FRY RIB-EYE STEAK

Preparation Time: 11 minutes

Cooking Time: 18 minutes

Servings: 2

Nutritional values:

- Calories: 470
- Fat: 31 g
- Carbohydrates: 23 g
- Proteins: 45 g

Ingredients:

- Lean rib eye steaks: 2 medium-sized
- Salt and freshly ground black pepper, to taste

Directions:

1. Let the air fry preheat at 400°F. pat dry steaks with paper towels.
2. Use any spice blend or just salt and pepper on steaks.

3. Generously on both sides of the steak.

4. Put steaks in the air fryer basket. Cook according to the rareness you want. Or cook for 14 minutes and flip after halftime.

5. Take out from the air fryer and let it rest for about 5 minutes.

6. Serve.

NORTH CAROLINA STYLE PORK CHOPS

Preparation Time: 9 minutes

Cooking Time: 18 minutes

Servings: 2

Nutritional values:

- Calories: 118 kcal
- Fat: 6.85 g
- Carbohydrates: 0 g
- Proteins: 13.1 g

Ingredients:

- 2 boneless pork chops
- 15 ml vegetable oil
- 25 g dark brown sugar, packaged
- 6 g Hungarian paprika
- 2 g ground mustard
- 2 g freshly ground black pepper

- 3 g onion powder
- 3 g garlic powder
- Salt and pepper to taste

Directions:

1. Preheat the air fryer for a few minutes at 180°C.
2. Cover the pork chops with oil.
3. Put all the spices and season the pork chops abundantly, almost as if you were making them breaded.
4. Place the pork chops in the preheated air fryer.
5. Select Steak and set the time to 10 minutes.
6. Remove the pork chops when it has finished cooking. Let it stand for 5 minutes and serve.

AIR FRYER BACON

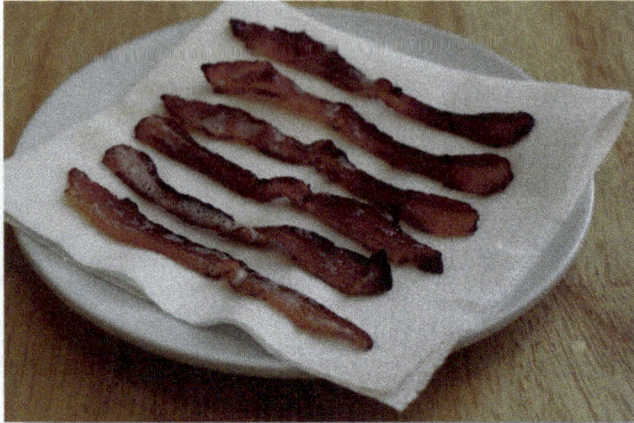

Preparation Time: 11 minutes

Cooking Time: 8 minutes

Servings: 4

Nutritional values:

- Calories: 91 kcal
- Carbohydrates: 0 g
- Fat: 8 g
- Proteins: 2 g

Ingredients:

- 11 bacon slices

Directions:

1. Divide the bacon in half, and place the first half in the air fryer.
2. Set the temperature at 401°F, and set the timer to 11 minutes.
3. Check it halfway through to see if anything needs to be rearranged.
4. Cook remainder of the time. Serve.

ROAST BEEF

Preparation Time: 6 minutes

Cooking Time: 48 minutes

Servings: 4

Nutritional values:

- Calories: 666 kcal
- Fat: 54 g
- Carbohydrates: 24 g
- Proteins: 43 g

Ingredients:

- 1 kg beef joint
- 1 tbsp. extra virgin olive oil
- Salt
- Pepper

Directions:

1. Rub the beef with extra virgin olive oil.

2. Season with pepper and salt.

3. Then place the seasoned beef onto the air fryer oven rotisserie and put it in place.

4. Adjust the timer to 45 minutes and the temperature to 380°F. Ensure the beef is rotating.

5. After 45 minutes, check the readiness, then slice the roast beef to pieces.

6. Serve

DIET BOILED RIBS

Preparation Time: 6 minutes

Cooking Time: 32 minutes

Servings: 4

Nutritional values:

- Calories 294
- Fat 17.9 g
- Carbohydrates 4.8 g
- Proteins 27.1 g

Ingredients:

- 400 g pork ribs
- 1 tsp. black pepper
- 1 g bay leaf
- 1 tsp. basil
- 1 white onion
- 1 carrot
- 1 tsp. cumin
- 700 ml water

Directions:

1. Cut the ribs on the portions and sprinkle it with black pepper.
2. Take a big saucepan and pour water into it.
3. Add the ribs and bay leaf.
4. Peel the onion and carrot and add them to the water with meat.
5. Sprinkle it with cumin and basil.
6. Cook it on medium heat in the air fryer for 30 minutes.

RUSSIAN STEAKS WITH NUTS AND CHEESE

Preparation Time: 8 minutes

Cooking Time: 22 minutes

Servings: 4

Nutritional values:

- Calories: 123.2 kcal
- Fat: 3.41 g
- Carbohydrates: 0 g
- Proteins: 20.9 g

Ingredients:

- 800 g minced pork
- 200 g cream cheese
- 50 g peeled walnuts
- 1 onion
- Salt
- Ground pepper

- 1 egg
- Breadcrumbs
- Extra virgin olive oil

Directions:

1. Put the onion cut into quarters in the Thermo mix glass and select 5 seconds speed 5.
2. Add the minced meat, cheese, egg, salt, and pepper.
3. Select 10 seconds, speed 5, turn left.
4. Add the chopped and peeled walnuts and select 4 seconds, turn left, speed 5.
5. Pass the dough to a bowl.
6. Make Russian steaks and go through breadcrumbs.
7. Paint the Russian fillets with extra virgin olive oil on both sides with a brush.
8. Put in the basket of the air fryer without stacking the Russian fillets.
9. Select 180°C and 15 minutes.

AIR FRYER SALMON FILLETS

Preparation Time: 5 minutes

Cooking Time: 16 minutes

Servings: 2

Nutritional values:

- Calories: 194 kcal
- Fat: 7 g
- Carbohydrates: 6 g
- Proteins: 25 g

Ingredients:

- ¼ cup low-fat Greek yogurt
- 2 salmon fillets
- 1 tbsp fresh dill (chopped)
- 1 lemon juice
- ½ garlic powder:
- Kosher salt and pepper

Directions:

1. Cut the lemon into slices and lay it at the bottom of the air fryer basket.

2. Season the salmon with kosher salt and pepper. Put salmon on top of lemons.

3. Let it cook at 330°For 15 minutes.

4. In the meantime, mix garlic powder, lemon juice, salt, pepper with yogurt and dill.

5. Serve the fish with sauce.

AIR FRYER FISH AND CHIPS

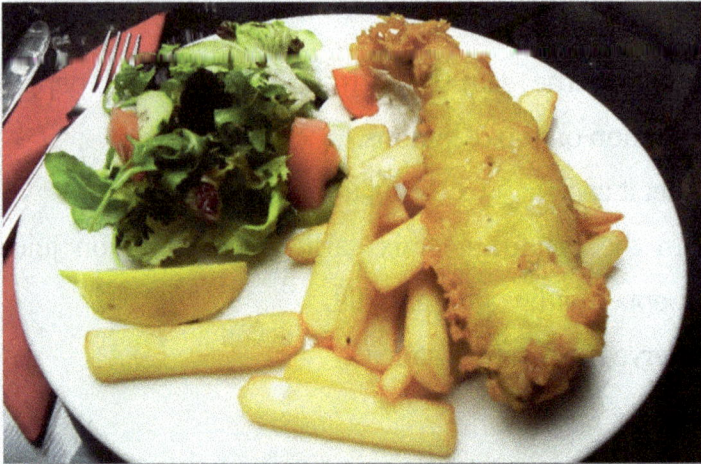

Preparation Time: 11 minutes

Cooking Time: 38 minutes

Servings: 4

Nutritional values:

- Calories: 409 kcal
- Fat: 11 g
- Carbohydrates: 44 g
- Proteins: 30 g

Ingredients:

- 4 cups any fish fillet
- flour: ¼ cup
- Whole wheat breadcrumbs: one cup
- One egg
- Oil: 2 tbsp.
- Potatoes
- Salt: 1 tsp.

Directions:

1. Cut the potatoes in fries. Then coat with oil and salt.
2. Cook in the air fryer for 20 minutes at 400°F, toss the fries halfway through.
3. In the meantime, coat fish in flour, then in the whisked egg, and finally in breadcrumbs mix.
4. Place the fish in the air fryer and let it cook at 330°F for 15 minutes.
5. Flip it halfway through, if needed.
6. Serve with tartar sauce and salad green.

GRILLED SALMON WITH LEMON

Preparation Time: 9 minutes

Cooking Time: 10 minutes

Servings: 4

Nutritional values:

- Calories: 211 kcal
- Fat: 9 g
- Carbohydrates: 4.9 g
- Proteins: 15 g

Ingredients:

- 2 tbsp. olive oil
- 2 salmon fillets
- Lemon juice
- 1/3 cup water
- 1/3 cup gluten-free light soy sauce
- 1/3 cup honey

- Scallion slices
- Cherry tomato
- Freshly ground black pepper, garlic powder, kosher salt to taste

Directions:

1. Season salmon with pepper and salt
2. In a bowl, mix honey, soy sauce, lemon juice, water, oil. Add salmon to this marinade and let it rest for at least two hours.
3. Let the air fryer preheat at 180°C
4. Place fish in the air fryer and cook for 8 minutes.
5. Move to a dish and top with scallion slices.

HARISSA ROASTED CORNISH GAME HENS

Preparation Time: 9 minutes

Cooking Time: 25-30 minutes

Servings: 4

Nutritional values:

- Calories: 412 kcal
- Fat: 32 g
- Carbohydrates: 5 g
- Proteins: 26 g

Ingredients:

Harissa:

- ½ cup olive oil
- 6 cloves garlic, minced
- 2 tbsp. smoked paprika

- 1 tbsp. ground coriander
- 1 tbsp. ground cumin
- 1 tsp. ground caraway
- 1 tsp. kosher salt
- ½ to 1 tsp. cayenne pepper

Hens:

- ½ cup yogurt
- 2 Cornish game hens, any giblets removed and split in half lengthwise

Directions:

1. For the harissa: In a medium microwave-safe bowl, combine the oil, garlic, paprika, coriander, cumin, caraway, salt, and cayenne. Microwave on high for 1 minute, stirring halfway through the cooking time. (You can also heat this on the stovetop until the oil is hot and bubbling. Or, if you must use your air fryer for everything, air fry it in the air fryer at 350°F (177°C) for 5 to 6 minutes, or until the pasta is heated through.)

2. For the hens: In a small bowl, combine 1 to 2 tbsp. of harissa and the yogurt. Whisk until well combined. Place the hen halves in a resealable plastic bag and pour the marinade over. Seal the bag and massage until all of the pieces are thoroughly coated. Marinate at room

temperature for 30 minutes or in the refrigerator for up to 24 hours.

3. Arrange the hen halves in a single layer in the air fryer basket. (If you have a smaller air fryer, you may have to cook this in two batches.) Roast at 400°F (204°C) for 20 minutes. Use a meat thermometer to ensure the game hens have reached an internal temperature of 165°F (74°C).

HONEY MUSTARD TURKEY BREAST

Preparation Time: 5 minutes

Cooking Time: 31 minutes

Servings: 4

Nutritional values:

- Calories: 526 kcal
- Fat: 22 g
- Carbohydrates: 18 g
- Proteins: 64 g

Ingredients:

- ¼ cup honey
- ¼ cup olive oil
- 1 tbsp. Dijon mustard
- 1 tbsp. butter, melted
- 2 tsp. minced garlic
- 1 tsp. salt

- ½ tsp. ground black pepper
- 2½ pound (1.1 kg) boneless turkey breast

Directions:

1. In a small bowl, whisk well to combine the honey, olive oil, Dijon mustard, butter, garlic, salt, and pepper.
2. Place the turkey breast in the air fryer basket, and brush with the honey mixture.
3. Bake at 400°F (204°C) for 20 minutes.
4. Remove the turkey breast, brush it with more of the honey mixture, and bake for an additional 10 minutes until golden.
5. Let the turkey rest for 5 to 10 minutes before slicing and serving.

SOUTH INDIAN PEPPER CHICKEN

Preparation Time: 22 minutes

Cooking Time: 18 minutes

Servings: 4

Nutritional values:

- Calories: 254 kcal
- Fat: 18 g
- Carbohydrates: 1 g
- Proteins: 22 g

Ingredients:

Spice Mix:

- 1 dried red chili or ½ tsp. dried red pepper flakes
- 1-inch piece cinnamon or cassia bark
- 1½ tsp. coriander seeds
- 1 tsp. fennel seeds
- 1 tsp. cumin seeds

- 1 tsp. black peppercorns
- ½ tsp. cardamom seeds
- ¼ tsp. ground turmeric
- 1 tsp. kosher salt

Chicken:

- 1 pound (454 g) boneless, skinless chicken thighs, cut crosswise into thirds
- 2 medium onions, cut into ½-inch-thick slices
- ¼ cup olive oil
- Cauliflower rice, steamed rice, or naan bread, for serving

Directions:

1. For the spice mix: Combine the dried chili, cinnamon, coriander, fennel, cumin, peppercorns, and cardamom in a clean coffee or spice grinder. Grind, shaking the grinder lightly so all the seeds and bits get into the blades, until the mixture is broken down to a fine powder. Stir in the turmeric and salt.

2. For the chicken: Place the chicken and onions in a resealable plastic bag. Add the oil and 1½ tbsp. of the spice mix. Seal the bag and massage until the chicken is well coated. Marinate at room temperature for 30 minutes or in the refrigerator for up to 24 hours.

3.   Place the chicken and onions in the air fryer basket. Bake at 350°F (177°C) for 10 minutes, stirring once halfway through the cooking time. Increase the temperature to 400°F (204°C) and bake for 5 minutes more. Use a meat thermometer to ensure the chicken has reached an internal temperature of 165°F (74°C).

4.   Serve with steamed rice, cauliflower rice, or naan.

MINI TURKEY MEATLOAVES

Preparation Time: 6 minutes

Cooking Time: 22 minutes

Servings: 4

Nutritional values:

- Calories: 142 kcal
- Fat: 5 g
- Carbohydrates: 3 g
- Proteins: 23 g

Ingredients:

- 1/3 cup minced onion
- ¼ cup grated carrot
- 2 garlic cloves, minced
- 2 tbsp. ground almonds
- 2 tsp. olive oil
- 1 tsp. dried marjoram
- 1 egg white
- ¾ pound (340 g) ground turkey breast

Directions:

1.   In a medium bowl, stir together the onion, carrot, garlic, almonds, olive oil, marjoram, and egg white.

2.   Add the ground turkey. With your hands, gently but— thoroughly mix until combined.

3.   Double 16 foil muffin cup liners to make 8 cups. Divide the turkey mixture evenly among the liners.

4.   Bake at 400°F (204°C) for 20 to 24 minutes, or until the meatloaves reach an internal temperature of 165°F (74°C) on a meat thermometer. Serve immediately.

CHEESE CHICKEN FRIES

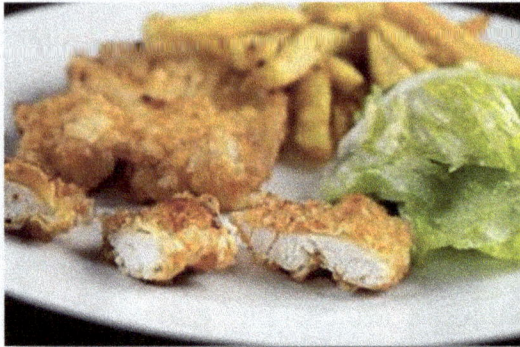

Preparation Time: 13 minutes

Cooking Time: 28 minutes

Servings: 4

Nutritional values:

- Calories: 242 kcal
- Fat: 6 g
- Carbohydrates: 3 g
- Proteins: 23 g

Ingredients:

- A pound of chicken (Cut into lengthy strips)

For the marinade:

- 1 tbsp. olive oil
- 1 tsp. mixed herbs
- ½ a tsp. red pepper flake
- 1/8 tsp. salt
- 1 tbsp. lemon juice
- For the garnish:
- A cup cheddar cheese (melted)

Directions:

1. Combine all the marinade ingredients into an empty bowl and mix properly.
2. Place chicken strips into a pot and boil them till partly cooked, then dip them into the prepared marinade and set aside.
3. Put the Air Fryer on and preheat for about 5 minutes at a temperature of 300°F. Put the chicken strips into the frying basket of the Air Fryer and cover basket.

4. Then set the temperature at 220°F for 20 minutes. Toss the fries about 3-4 times during the cooking process to ensure even cooking.

5. Just before the cooking time elapses, spread the coriander leaves on fries. Then take fries out, serving them with the melted cheese as topping.

CHICKEN FINGERS

Preparation Time: 15 minutes

Cooking Time: 22 minutes

Servings: 4

Nutritional values:

- Calories: 142 kcal
- Fat: 5 g
- Carbohydrates: 3 g
- Proteins: 23 g

Ingredients:

- 2 tsp. red pepper flakes
- 1 pound boneless skinless chicken breasts (cut into strips)
- 2 cupsful dry breadcrumbs
- 2 tsp. oregano

For Marinade:

- 2 tsp. salt
- 6 tbsp. corn flour

- 1 and ½ tbsp. of ginger-garlic paste
- 1 tsp. black pepper
- 4 tbsp. fresh lemon juice
- 1 tsp. chili powder
- 5 eggs

Directions:

1. Put all ingredients required for the marinade into a bowl and mix adequately. Put the stripped chicken breasts into the bowl and refrigerate overnight to marinate sufficiently.

2. Now combine the 1 tsp. red pepper flakes, 2 tsp. oregano, and 2 cups breadcrumbs in an empty bowl and mix properly. Coat marinated chicken strips in breadcrumb mix and cover them with a food wrap till ready to cook.

3. Switch on your Air Fryer and preheat at a temperature of 160°F for a time frame of 5 minutes. Then put the chicken strips into the basket and close. Allow chicken strips to cook for a further 15 minutes at the same temperature, tossing them properly at intervals to ensure an even fry.

4. Dish into plates and serve.

JUICY KEBAB

Preparation Time: 15 minutes

Cooking Time: 32 minutes

Servings: 8

Nutritional values:

- Calories: 282 kcal
- Fat: 5 g
- Carbohydrates: 4 g
- Proteins: 21 g

Ingredients:

- 4 small onions (diced)
- 5 green chilies (coarsely chopped)
- 2 pounds chicken breasts (cut into cubes)
- 4 tbsp. fresh mint leaves (chopped)
- 3 tbsp. cream
- 3 tbsp. capsicum peppers
- 1 and ½ tbsp. of ginger paste
- 1 and ½ tsp. salt

- 2 garlic cloves (crushed)
- 2 tbsp. powdered coriander
- 3 tsp. fresh lemon juice
- 2 tsp. garam masala
- 3 eggs
- 4 tbsp. cilantro
- 2 tbsp. peanut flour

Directions:

1. Combine all the dry ingredients into an empty bowl and mix properly. Add a little water and mix the dry ingredients properly to produce a fine paste. Put eggs into a bowl and beat them using a whisk, adding a little salt.

2. Immerse the chicken cubes in the mixture made, coating each completely and then refrigerating them for an hour.

3. Turn on the Air Fryer and preheat for 5 minutes at 250°F. Take out the fry basket and lay kebabs inside, spacing them appropriately. Cook kebabs at 290F for 25 minutes, flipping after a while to ensure an even cook.

4. Serve kebab with mint or basil chutney.

BRUSSELS SPROUTS

Preparation Time: 5 minutes

Cooking Time: 10 minutes

Servings: 2

Nutritional values:

- Calories: 88
- Fat: 4.4 g
- Carbohydrates: 11 g
- Proteins: 3.9 g

Ingredients:

- 2 cups Brussels sprouts
- ¼ tsp. sea salt
- 1 tbsp. olive oil
- 1 tbsp. apple cider vinegar

Directions:

1. Switch on the air fryer, insert fryer basket, grease it with olive oil, then shut with its lid, set the fryer at 400°F and preheat for 5 minutes.

2. Meanwhile, cut the sprouts lengthwise into ¼-inch thick pieces, add them in a bowl, add remaining ingredients and toss until well coated.

3. Open the fryer, add sprouts in it, close with its lid and cook for 10 minutes until crispy and cooked, shaking halfway through the frying.

4. When the air fryer beeps, open its lid, transfer sprouts onto a serving plate, and serve.

GREEN BEANS

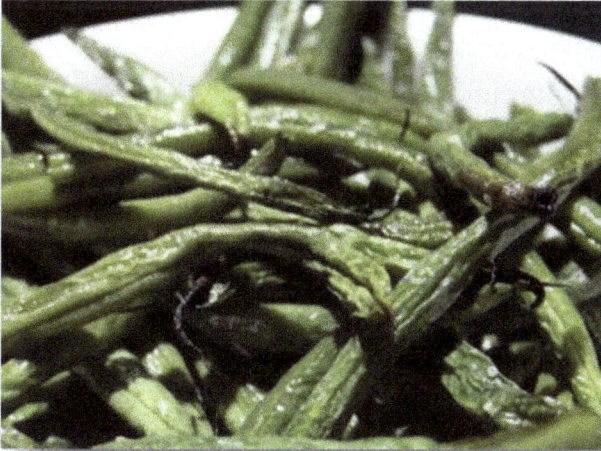

Preparation Time: 5 minutes

Cooking Time: 13 minutes

Servings: 4

Nutritional values:

- Calories: 45 kcal
- Fat: 1 g
- Carbohydrates: 7 g
- Proteins: 2 g

Ingredients:

- 1-pound green beans
- ¾ tsp. garlic powder
- ¾ tsp. ground black pepper
- 1 ¼ tsp. salt
- ½ tsp. paprika

Directions:

1. Switch on the air fryer, insert fryer basket, grease it with olive oil, then shut with its lid, set the fryer at 400°F and preheat for 5 minutes.

2. Meanwhile, place beans in a bowl, spray generously with olive oil, sprinkle with garlic powder, black pepper, salt, and paprika and toss until well coated.

3. Open the fryer, add green beans in it, close with its lid and cook for 8 minutes until nicely golden and crispy, shaking halfway through the frying.

4. When the air fryer beeps, open its lid, transfer green beans onto a serving plate and serve.

ASPARAGUS SOUP

Preparation Time: 10 minutes

Cooking Time: 20 minutes

Servings: 4

Nutritional values:

- Calories: 208 kcal
- Fat: 16 g
- Carbohydrates: 13 g
- Proteins: 6 g

Ingredients:

- 1 avocado, peeled, pitted, cubed
- 12 ounces asparagus
- ½ tsp. ground black pepper
- 1 tsp. garlic powder
- 1 tsp. sea salt
- 2 tbsp. olive oil, divided
- ½ lemon, juiced
- 2 cups vegetable stock

Directions:

1.   Switch on the air fryer, insert fryer basket, grease it with olive oil, then shut with its lid, set the fryer at 425°F and preheat for 5 minutes.

2.   Meanwhile, place asparagus in a shallow dish, drizzle with 1 tbsp. oil, sprinkle with garlic powder, salt, and black pepper, and toss until well mixed.

3.   Open the fryer, add asparagus in it, close with its lid and cook for 10 minutes until nicely golden and roasted, shaking halfway through the frying.

4.   When the air fryer beeps, open its lid and transfer asparagus to a food processor.

5.   Add remaining ingredients into a food processor and pulse until well combined and smooth.

6.   Tip the soup in a saucepan, pour in water if the soup is too thick and heat it over medium-low heat for 5 minutes until thoroughly heated.

7.   Ladle soup into bowls and serve.

CRUNCHY BRUSSELS SPROUTS

Preparation Time: 9 minutes

Cooking Time: 5 minutes

Servings: 2

Nutritional values:

- Calories: 92 kcal
- Fat: 3.1 g
- Carbohydrates: 12.1 g
- Proteins: 5.2 g

Ingredients:

- 1 tsp. avocado oil
- 1/2 tsp. black pepper (ground)
- 1/2 tsp salt
- Ten ounces Brussels sprouts (halved)
- One-third tsp. balsamic vinegar

Directions:

1. Heat the air fryer at 175°C.

2. Mix salt, pepper, and oil together in a bowl. Add the sprouts and toss.

3. Fry the Brussels sprouts in the air fryer for five minutes.

BUFFALO CAULIFLOWER

Preparation Time: 11 minutes

Cooking Time: 30 minutes

Servings: 4

Nutritional values:

- Calories: 190
- Fat: 12 g
- Carbohydrates: 2.3 g
- Proteins: 12.3 g

Ingredients:

- 1 large cauliflower
- 1 cup flour
- ¼ tsp. each
- Chili powder
- Cayenne pepper
- Paprika
- 1 cup soy milk
- 2 tbsp. butter

- 2 garlic cloves (minced)
- ½ cup cayenne pepper sauce
- One serving cooking spray

Directions:

1. Cut the cauliflower into small pieces. Rinse under cold water and drain.
2. Mix flour, chili powder, cayenne, and paprika in a bowl. Add the milk slowly to make a thick batter.
3. Add the pieces of cauliflower in the batter and coat well.
4. Cook the cauliflower in the air fryer for twenty minutes. Toss the cauliflower and cook again for ten minutes.
5. Take a saucepan and heat the butter in it. Add garlic and hot sauce. Boil the sauce mixture and simmer for two minutes.
6. Transfer the cauliflower to a large bowl and pour the prepared sauce over the cooked cauliflower. Toss for combining.
7. Serve hot.

STUFFED MUSHROOMS

Preparation Time: 12 minutes

Cooking Time: 10-15 minutes

Servings: 6

Nutritional values:

- Calories: 42 kcal
- Fat: 1.2 g
- Carbohydrates: 2.9 g
- Proteins: 3.1 g

Ingredients:

- Fifteen button mushrooms
- 1 tsp. olive oil
- 1/8 tsp. salt
- ½ tsp. black pepper (crushed)
- 1/3 tsp. balsamic vinegar

For the filling:

- ¼ cup each

- Bell pepper
- Onion
- 2 tbsp. cilantro (chopped)
- 1 tbsp. jalapeno (chopped finely)
- ½ cupmozzarella cheese (grated)
- 1 tsp. coriander (ground)
- ¼ tsp. each
- Paprika
- Salt

Directions:

1. Use a damp cloth for cleaning the mushrooms. Remove the stems for making the caps hollow.
2. Take a bowl and season the mushroom caps with salt, oil, balsamic vinegar, and black pepper.
3. Take another bowl and mix the ingredients for the filling.
4. Use a spoon to fill the mushroom caps. Press the filling in the mushroom using the backside of the spoon.
5. Cook the mushrooms in the air fryer for ten minutes.
6. Serve hot.

SWEET POTATOES WITH BAKED TAQUITOS

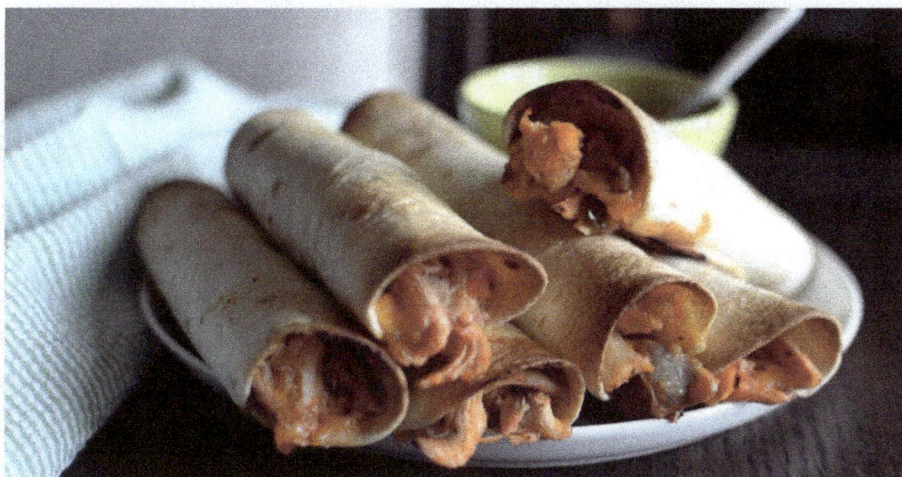

Preparation Time: 5 minutes

Cooking Time: 20 minutes

Servings: 5

Nutritional values:

- Calories: 112 kcal
- Fat: 1.6 g
- Carbohydrates: 19.3 g
- Proteins: 5.2 g

Ingredients:

- 1 sweet potato (cut in half an inch)
- 2 tsps. canola oil
- ½ cup yellow onion (chopped)
- 1 garlic clove (minced)
- 2 cups black beans (rinsed)
- 1 chipotle pepper (chopped)
- ½ tsp. each
- Paprika
- Cumin
- Chili powder
- Maple syrup
- 1/8 tsp. salt
- 3 tbsp. water
- 10 corn tortillas

Directions:

1. Place the pieces of sweet potatoes in an air fryer and toss them with some oil. Cook for twelve minutes. Make sure you shake the basket in between.

2. Take a skillet and heat some oil in it. Add the garlic and onions. Sauté for five minutes until the onions are translucent.

3. Add chipotle pepper, beans, paprika, cumin, chili powder, maple syrup, and salt. Add two tbsp. water and mix all the ingredients.

4. Add cooked potatoes and mix well.

5. Warm the corn tortillas in a skillet.

6. Put two tbsp. of beans and potato mixture in a row across the corn tortillas. Grab one end of the corn tortillas and roll them. Tuck the end under the mixture of sweet potato and beans.

7. Place the taquitos with the seam side down in the basket. Spray the taquitos with some oil. Air fry the prepared taquitos for ten minutes.

8. Serve hot.

CAULIFLOWER CURRY

Preparation Time: 8 minutes

Cooking Time: 15 minutes

Servings: 3

Nutritional values:

- Calories: 160 kcal
- Proteins: 5.2 g
- Carbohydrates: 27.2 g
- Fat: 3.1 g

Ingredients:

- 1 cup vegetable stock
- ¾ cup coconut milk (light)
- 2 tsps. curry powder
- 1 tsp. garlic puree
- ½ tsp. turmeric
- 12 ounces cauliflower (cut in florets)
- 1 and a half cup sweet corn kernels
- 3 spring onions (sliced)

- Salt

For the topping:

- Lime wedges
- Two tbsp. dried cranberries

Directions:

1. Heat your air fryer at 190°C.
2. Mix all ingredients in a large bowl. Combine well.
3. Transfer the cauliflower mixture to the air fryer basket.
4. Cook for fifteen minutes. Give it a mix in the middle.

GINGER CHEESECAKE

Preparation Time: 2 hours and 30 minutes

Cooking Time: 20-25 minutes

Servings: 6

Nutritional values:

- Calories: 195 kcal
- Fat: 18 g
- Carbohydrates: 2 g
- Proteins: 4 g

Ingredients:

- 2 tbsp. butter
- ½ cup ginger cookies
- 16 oz. cream cheese
- 2 eggs
- ½ cup sugar
- 1 tbsp. rum

- ½ tbsp. vanilla extract
- ½ tbsp. nutmeg

Directions:

1. Spread pan with the butter and sprinkle cookie crumbs on the bottom.
2. Whisk cream cheese with rum, vanilla, nutmeg, and eggs, beat properly and sprinkle the cookie crumbs.
3. Put in the air fryer and cook at 340°F for 20 minutes.
4. Allow cheesecake to cool in the fridge for 2 hours before slicing.
5. Serve.

COCOA COOKIES

Preparation Time: 10 minutes

Cooking Time: 15-20 minutes

Servings: 12

Nutritional values:

- Calories: 185 kcal
- Fat: 19 g
- Carbohydrates: 6 g
- Proteins: 4 g

Ingredients:

- 6 oz. coconut oil
- 6 eggs
- 3 oz. cocoa powder
- 2 tbsp. vanilla
- ½ tbsp. baking powder
- 4 oz. cream cheese
- 5 tbsp. sugar

Directions:

1.   Mix in eggs with coconut oil, baking powder, cocoa powder, cream cheese, vanilla in a blender and sway and turn using a mixer.

2.   Get it into a lined baking dish and into the fryer at 320°F and bake for 14 minutes.

3.   Split cookie sheet into rectangles.

4.   Serve.

SPECIAL BROWNIES

Preparation Time: 10 minutes

Cooking Time: 38 minutes

Servings: 4

Nutritional values:

- Calories: 129 kcal
- Fat: 11 g
- Carbohydrates: 8 g
- Proteins: 2 g

Ingredients:

- 1 egg
- 1/3 cup cocoa powder
- 1/3 cup sugar
- 7 tbsp. butter
- ½ tbsp. vanilla extract
- ¼ cup white flour
- ¼ cup walnuts
- ½ tbsp. baking powder

- 1 tbsp. peanut butter

Directions:

1. Warm pan with 6 tbsp. butter and the sugar over medium heat, turn, cook for 5 minutes, move to a bowl, put salt, egg, cocoa powder, vanilla extract, walnuts, baking powder and flour, turn mix properly and into a pan.

2. Mix peanut butter with one tbsp. butter in a bowl, heat in the microwave for some seconds, turn properly and sprinkle brownies blend over.

3. Put in the air fryer and bake at 320°F and bake for 17 minutes.

4. Allow brownies to cool, cut.

5. Serve.

BLUEBERRY SCONES

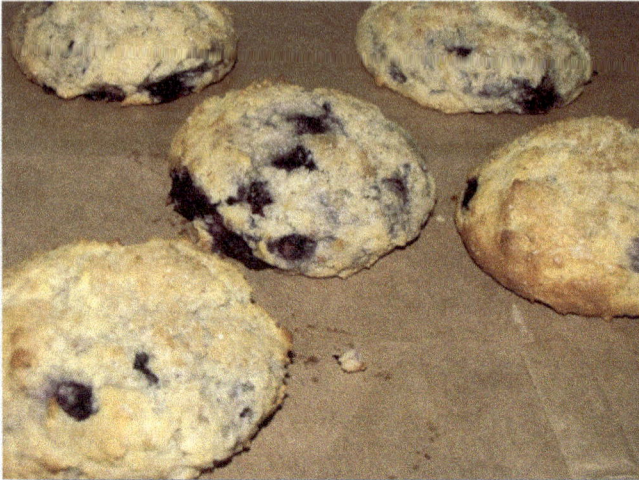

Preparation Time: 20 minutes

Cooking Time: 15-20 minutes

Servings: 10

Nutritional values:

- Calories: 195 kcal
- Fat: 16 g
- Carbohydrates: 8 g
- Proteins: 4 g

Ingredients:

- 1 cup white flour
- 1 cup blueberries
- 2 eggs
- ½ cup heavy cream
- ½ cup butter
- 5 tbsp. sugar
- 2 tbsp. vanilla extract
- 2 tbsp. baking powder

Directions:

1. Mix in flour, baking powder, salt and blueberries in a bowl and turn.
2. Mix heavy cream with vanilla extract, sugar, butter, and eggs and turn properly.
3. Blend the 2 mixtures, squeeze till the dough is ready, obtain 10 triangles from the mix, put on the baking sheet into the air fryer and cook them at 320°F for 10 minutes.
4. Serve cold.

CHOCOLATE COOKIES

Preparation Time: 10 minutes

Cooking Time: 26 minutes

Servings: 12

Nutritional values:

- Calories: 147 kcal
- Fat: 20 g
- Carbohydrates: 4 g
- Proteins: 3 g

Ingredients:

- 1 tbsp. vanilla extract
- ½ cup butter
- 1 egg
- 4 tbsp. sugar
- 2 cups flour
- ½ cup unsweetened chocolate chips

Directions:

1. Warm pan with butter over medium heat, turn and cook for 1 minute.
2. Mix in egg with sugar and vanilla extract in a bowl and turn properly.
3. Put flour, melted butter and half of the chocolate chips, and turn.
4. Move to a pan, sprinkle the remaining chocolate chips over, put in the fryer at 330°F and bake for 25 minutes.
5. Serve slices when cold.

www.ingramcontent.com/pod-product-compliance
Lightning Source LLC
Chambersburg PA
CBHW050745030426
42336CB00012B/1671